TABLE OF CONTENT

CHAPTER 1. UNDERSTANDING REFLEXOLOGY AND FERTILITY: INTRODUCE THE CONCEPT OF REFLEXOLOGY AND ITS POTENTIAL IMPACT ON FERTILITY. EXPLAIN HOW REFLEXOLOGY WORKS, ITS UNDERLYING PRINCIPLES, AND HOW IT CAN INFLUENCE REPRODUCTIVE HEALTH.

CHAPTER 2. MAPPING THE REPRODUCTIVE REFLEX POINTS: EXPLORE THE SPECIFIC REFLEX POINTS ON THE FEET AND HANDS THAT ARE ASSOCIATED WITH THE REPRODUCTIVE ORGANS AND SYSTEMS. PROVIDE DETAILED EXPLANATIONS AND DIAGRAMS TO HELP READERS LOCATE THESE POINTS FOR EFFECTIVE SELF-CARE.

CHAPTER 3. BALANCING HORMONES THROUGH REFLEXOLOGY: DISCUSS THE HORMONAL IMBALANCES THAT CAN AFFECT FERTILITY AND EXPLAIN HOW REFLEXOLOGY CAN HELP REGULATE HORMONES. PROVIDE REFLEXOLOGY TECHNIQUES

AND ROUTINES AIMED AT TARGETING HORMONE-PRODUCING GLANDS.

CHAPTER 4. STRESS REDUCTION AND FERTILITY ENHANCEMENT: EXAMINE THE RELATIONSHIP BETWEEN STRESS AND FERTILITY CHALLENGES. PRESENT REFLEXOLOGY AS A RELAXATION TECHNIQUE THAT CAN ALLEVIATE STRESS, REDUCE ANXIETY, AND CREATE A CONDUCIVE ENVIRONMENT FOR CONCEPTION.

CHAPTER 5. ENHANCING BLOOD FLOW TO THE REPRODUCTIVE ORGANS: HIGHLIGHT THE IMPORTANCE OF PROPER BLOOD CIRCULATION FOR REPRODUCTIVE HEALTH. DESCRIBE REFLEXOLOGY TECHNIQUES THAT STIMULATE BLOOD FLOW TO THE PELVIC REGION, THEREBY IMPROVING THE SUPPLY OF NUTRIENTS AND OXYGEN TO REPRODUCTIVE ORGANS.

CHAPTER 6. SUPPORTING MEN'S FERTILITY THROUGH REFLEXOLOGY: ADDRESS MALE FERTILITY ISSUES AND HOW REFLEXOLOGY CAN BENEFIT MEN'S REPRODUCTIVE HEALTH. DISCUSS REFLEXOLOGY POINTS THAT TARGET THE MALE

Reflexology for fertility

How to Get Pregnant Quickly:

Preparing Your Body for

Pregnancy With Reflexology

Dan Phillips PhD

~DEDICATION~

~LARRY~

For your unwavering support, encouragement, and friendship. Your presence in my life has been a constant source of inspiration. Thank you for your invaluable kindness and belief in my journey. This book is a token of appreciation for your enduring friendship and steadfast encouragement.

REPRODUCTIVE SYSTEM AND PROVIDE GUIDANCE FOR COUPLES TO PRACTICE TOGETHER.

CHAPTER 7. REFLEXOLOGY FOR ASSISTED REPRODUCTIVE TECHNIQUES (ART): EXPLORE HOW REFLEXOLOGY CAN COMPLEMENT MEDICAL INTERVENTIONS SUCH AS IN VITRO FERTILIZATION (IVF) OR INTRAUTERINE INSEMINATION (IUI). OFFER REFLEXOLOGY PRACTICES TO PREPARE THE BODY FOR THESE PROCEDURES AND ENHANCE THEIR SUCCESS RATES.

CHAPTER 8. LIFESTYLE AND NUTRITION TIPS ALONGSIDE REFLEXOLOGY: PROVIDE HOLISTIC ADVICE BY INTEGRATING REFLEXOLOGY WITH HEALTHY LIFESTYLE CHOICES AND NUTRITION. SHARE RECOMMENDATIONS FOR OPTIMAL DIETS, EXERCISE ROUTINES, AND RELAXATION TECHNIQUES TO SUPPORT OVERALL FERTILITY IN CONJUNCTION WITH REFLEXOLOGY PRACTICES.

CHAPTER 1

**Understanding Reflexology and
Fertility: Introduce the concept of
reflexology and its potential impact
on fertility. Explain how reflexology
works, its underlying principles,
and how it can influence
reproductive health.**

Within the field of complementary
and alternative medicine, reflexology
is a particularly noteworthy practice
that has drawn interest from those
looking for all-natural remedies for a
range of health problems, including

infertility. By illuminating the fundamental ideas and possible effects of reflexology on reproductive health, this chapter seeks to disentangle the complex relationship between reflexology and fertility.

The Idea of Reflexology: A Synopsis

The healing art of reflexology has been around for thousands of years, having its roots in the ancient cultures of Egypt, China, and India. Reflexology's basic tenet is that particular organs, systems, and glands in the body are represented by particular reflex sites on the hands, feet, and ears. It is claimed that these reflex sites are connected by energy channels, and that energy blockages can be cleared by applying pressure to these spots, hence supporting the body's inherent healing and restoring capacity.

Impact on Fertility Possible

Reflexology has been accepted for its ability to treat a variety of illnesses, but in the last several years, its function in boosting fertility has attracted a lot of notice. Millions of couples worldwide struggle with infertility, which is defined as the inability to conceive after a year of unprotected sexual activity.

Reflexology provides a non-invasive, all-encompassing strategy in this regard that seeks to address the psychological as well as the physical aspects that may be involved in fertility difficulties.

The Function of Reflexology

The underlying tenet of reflexology is that the body is an integrated whole, with all of its parts interacting and impacting the total. According to reflexologists, when particular reflex sites are stimulated with light pressure, nerve signals are sent to the associated organs or systems, encouraging stress relief, better blood circulation, and relaxation. Reproductive organs such the ovaries, fallopian tubes, uterus, and prostate in males are thought to benefit from the use of reflexology techniques to the reproductive reflex points in the context of fertility. The goal of reflexology is to establish an environment that is favorable to conception by encouraging relaxation and improving blood flow to specific areas.

Key Players in Reproductive Reflex Points

The reproductive reflex points are essential to reflexology for fertility. These spots are thought to have a direct relationship to the reproductive systems and organs and are placed strategically on the hands and feet. For example, the inner sides of the feet correlate to the reflex points for the uterus and ovaries, whereas the inside of the heel corresponds to the reflex point for the prostate. Reflexologists carefully lay out these ideas, using both modern science and traditional knowledge to inform their work.

The Link Between Mind and Body

Beyond its physical components, reflexology acknowledges the close connection between the body and mind. Problems with fertility are frequently made worse by emotional, psychological, and stressful causes. The method of relaxation used in reflexology is consistent with this concept. Through the use of soothing touch, reflexology works to activate the parasympathetic nervous system, which lowers stress levels and promotes relaxation. In turn, this may benefit the balance of hormones and general reproductive health.

Inquiry into Science and Reflexology

Though holistic devotees may find resonance in the concepts of reflexology, skeptics frequently seek scientific validation. Numerous studies have started to look into the possible advantages of reflexology for reproductive health, but more research is still required. Psychoneuroimmunology research indicates that stress reduction by reflexology and other therapies may impact immunological responses and hormone control, which may have an indirect effect on fertility. Furthermore, after receiving reflexology treatments, some studies have shown that women with polycystic ovarian syndrome (PCOS) experienced improved menstrual regularity and decreased pain.

Result: A Way to Increase Fertility

In a world where contemporary medicine provides a range of interventions for fertility issues, reflexology shows up as an additional path that takes into account both the mental and physical health of individuals and couples as well as the physical aspects of reproductive health. Reflexology offers a comprehensive approach to fertility improvement by taking into account the complex relationship between mind and body and the body's inherent healing mechanisms. This book will go deeper into the useful methods and approaches that use reflexology to help the body get ready for pregnancy as the chapters go by, giving those who are preparing to become parents a sense of empowerment and hope.

CHAPTER 2

Mapping the Reproductive Reflex Points: Explore the specific reflex points on the feet and hands that are associated with the reproductive organs and systems. Provide detailed explanations and diagrams to help readers locate these points for effective self-care.

Within the field of alternative therapies and holistic medicine, reflexology has become a highly effective technique for fostering bodily balance and well-being. Reflexology, which has its roots in both historical customs and contemporary anatomy, targets particular pressure spots on the hands and feet to stimulate healing responses in the relevant organs and systems. This thorough guide's second chapter sets out to demystify the complex web of reproductive reflex points, illuminating their importance and encouraging readers to take care of their reproductive health on their own.

The Detailed Chart: An Assisted Tour of Stress Points

The idea that the hands and feet reflect the internal architecture of the body is fundamental to reflexology. Through the deft application of these reflex spots, people can initiate advantageous physiological reactions and support the body's natural healing processes. We explore the reproductive reflex point map in this chapter, providing a road map for self-care.

Understanding the Connection: It's important to understand the body's vast connection before diving into the details of reproductive reflex points. The idea of zones, in which different parts of the hand and foot correlate to different organs and systems, is a concept used by reflexologists. These zones contain the reproductive reflex points, which serve as portals to vitality and equilibrium.

Locating the Reflex spots: The book is accompanied by comprehensive diagrams that walk readers through the process of identifying reproductive reflex spots. These points are mostly located on the inner arch of the feet, and they represent the uterus, ovaries, and pelvis. Approaching the hands, the matching reflex points are located along the inner border, in line with the foot alignment. Clear illustrations combined with step-by-step directions enable readers to confidently traverse this healing terrain.

Points of Vitality: In the field of reproductive reflexology, vital points are essential for fostering well-being and addressing certain issues. The "Uterus Oasis," which is tucked away inside the foot's inner arch, is one such location. It is thought that stimulating this spot will improve general reproductive health and ease menstrual discomfort. In the same way, the "Sacral Sanctuary," which is located close to the base of the thumb, provides a technique to balance the sacral chakra and promote emotional stability. The vast potential that is just under their feet, or rather, at their fingertips, is made more apparent to readers by these thorough explanations.

Anatomy and Energetic Views: Investigating the Nexus

A thorough comprehension of reproductive reflex sites requires investigation from both anatomical and energetic perspectives.

Anatomical Insights: the relationship between the reflex points and reproductive organs is not coincidental; rather, it stems from a common embryonic ancestry. Different tissues differentiate into unique structures as the body grows, yet connections between them are preserved. This embryological link is used by reflexologists to explain why reflexology works so well. Through the activation of a reflex point, practitioners hope to improve nerve impulses, blood flow, and energy exchange in the associated organ or system, promoting health and vitality.

Energetic Harmony: Traditional Chinese medicine and other holistic traditions are incorporated into reflexology concepts in addition to the physical aspect. Meridians, or energetic routes, are believed to run through the body and facilitate the movement of life force, or "qi." These meridians connect at reproductive reflex locations, facilitating the harmonizing of energy flow. This dual viewpoint, which combines energy dynamics and embodied anatomy, provides a more comprehensive understanding of the complex interplay between the reproductive organs and reflex sites.

Self-Care Empowerment: Unlocking the Healing Potential

With this knowledge and the reflexology tenets as their guide, readers are well-prepared to set out on a path of holistic healing and self-care.

The Art of Stimulation: Chapter 2 explores the methods of applying pressure, varying its duration, and varying its rhythm to stimulate reproductive reflex sites. Using the thumbs, fingers, or specialized reflexology instruments, readers learn how to use their body's natural understanding to support reproductive health.

correcting Imbalances: Reproductive reflexology is a technique for correcting imbalances in addition to being used to maintain wellness. In the expert hands of reflexology practitioners, irregular menstrual cycles, hormonal irregularities, and stress-related reproductive disorders may find a possible ally. By applying pressure to particular reflex spots, people may be able to reduce pain and regain their balance.

Conclusion

This thorough guide's second chapter explains how to comprehend and work with reproductive reflex points, a field where traditional knowledge collides with contemporary anatomy and energy theory. By means of thorough explanations, striking illustrations, and perceptive stories, readers are enabled to unleash the potential of reflexology for the health of their reproductive systems. The complex network of connections between the hands, feet, and reproductive organs becomes a canvas for nourishing vitality, harmony, and balance as they set out on this path of self-care and inquiry.

CHAPTER 3

Balancing Hormones Through Reflexology: Discuss the hormonal imbalances that can affect fertility and explain how reflexology can help regulate hormones. Provide reflexology techniques and routines aimed at targeting hormone-producing glands.

The complex dance of the human reproductive system depends heavily on hormonal balance. Unbalanced hormones can interfere with ovulation, regular menstruation, and overall reproductive health, all of which can lead to infertility. This chapter explores the intricacies of hormonal balance and how reflexology can be used as a complementary therapy to balance hormones and encourage ideal conception.

The Hormone Symphony: Fertility Effects

Hormones are transmitters that help the body coordinate many physiological functions, including reproduction. A number of things, including stress, a poor diet, inactivity, and underlying medical issues, can lead to hormonal imbalances. Thyroid issues and polycystic ovarian syndrome (PCOS) are two conditions that can severely disrupt hormonal balance and exacerbate fertility problems. Anovulation, or the absence of ovulation, irregular menstrual cycles, and luteal phase defects are common signs of hormonal disorders that prevent pregnancy.

Reflexology's Relationship

The basis of reflexology is the idea that the body's reflex sites correspond to different organs and systems, including glands that produce hormones. Reflexology works by applying pressure to certain reflex spots with the intention of stimulating nerve pathways, which in turn affect the associated glands. Techniques used in reflexology can be tailored to support the appropriate functioning of these glands within the framework of hormonal balance.

The Hormone-Producing Glands and Reflex Points

Vascular Gland: The pituitary gland, sometimes called the "master gland," regulates the release of hormones from other endocrine glands. Approaches to reflexology that concentrate on the head, particularly the big toes, may affect the activity and regulation of hormones by the pituitary gland.

Gonadal Gland: The thyroid gland, which is located in the neck, is essential for controlling hormones and metabolism. The stimulation of reflexology points on the feet that relate to the neck region may help to support thyroid function.

- Glands Adrenal: Cortisol and other stress-related chemicals are produced by the adrenal glands. By using reflexology techniques to target the adrenal reflex sites, one can indirectly impact hormone balance through stress management.

Testes and Ovaries: Reflex points on the hands and feet correspond to the reproductive organs itself. Targeting these reflex sites using reflexology techniques may promote better testicular and ovarian function, which helps maintain hormone balance.

- Dermatome: Blood sugar levels are impacted by insulin, which is produced by the pancreas. Pancreas reflex points are the focus of reflexology procedures that may help support insulin sensitivity and metabolic balance.

Combining Reflexology with Hormone Balancing

1. System of the Endocrine System: In this complete reflexology routine, pressure is applied to the reflex points that correlate to the glands responsible for endocrine function. It seeks to support hormonal balance by

energizing and balancing the entire endocrine system.

2. Regulation of the Menstrual Cycle: A specific reflexology regimen can be created to target the ovaries, uterus, and pituitary gland for women who experience irregular menstrual periods. The goal of this sequence is to promote normal menstrual cycles and ovulation.

3. Strategies for Stress Reduction: Hormonal imbalances may be exacerbated by prolonged stress. Stress management and hormonal stability can be supported by reflexology techniques that

concentrate on stress-relieving reflex sites, such as those connected to the adrenal glands.

The Comprehensive Method for Managing Hormones

It's crucial to remember that reflexology cannot treat serious hormone imbalances or medical disorders on its own. On the other hand, it can function as an adjunctive method to traditional medical treatments. In order to balance hormones and improve fertility, reflexology promotes relaxation, improves blood circulation, and supports the body's natural healing processes.

Final Thought: Strengthening Hormonal Balance

A critical and complex part of reproductive health is hormone balance. Through the use of particular reflex sites, reflexology offers a novel approach to supporting hormonal homeostasis by altering hormone-producing glands. Individuals and couples can optimize their chances of conception and restore hormonal harmony by incorporating customized reflexology therapies into their health practice. This chapter starts the powerful adventure of using reflexology to balance hormones and improve fertility, as the next chapters will go into more detail on doable methods and practices.

CHAPTER 4

Stress Reduction and Fertility Enhancement: Examine the relationship between stress and fertility challenges. Present reflexology as a relaxation technique that can alleviate stress, reduce anxiety, and create a conducive environment for conception.

The complicated relationship between stress and reproductive function is a key component of human health and well-being. The significant impact of stress on problems with reproduction has come into greater prominence as science progresses. Delves into this sensitive nexus, Chapter 4 clarifies the unmistakable connection between reproductive problems and stress. It also presents reflexology as a powerful relaxing method that can be used to ease tension, lessen anxiety, and create an atmosphere that is favorable to conception.

The Stress-Fertility Puzzle: Dissecting the Details

With its fast-paced lifestyle and never-ending demands, modern living has elevated stress to the top of the health concern list. Chronic stress upsets the body's delicate hormonal balances and physiological processes by cascading throughout the body. The implications of the stress response can extend well within the domain of reproduction.

The Hormonal Orchestra: Prolonged stress causes the release of cortisol, which is sometimes called the "stress hormone." The precise balance of reproductive hormones, such as those governing ovulation, menstruation, and the menstrual cycle, may be upset by this spike in cortisol. When a woman's body fails to produce enough hormones to conceive, she may experience irregular periods, anovulation, or even decreased ovarian function.

The Mind-Body Connection: Stress affects hormones and creates a complex web of interconnectedness between the mind and body. Blood flow to the reproductive organs can be reduced by blood vessel constriction brought on by stress and anxiety. The likelihood of successful fertilization and implantation decreases in this weakened setting. Furthermore, the psychological effects of stress can lower sexual desire and libido, which further reduces the likelihood of conception.

Reflexology: A Way to De-stress and Boost Fertility

In light of this complex interaction between stress and fertility, reflexology stands out as a ray of hope by providing a comprehensive strategy for relaxation and overall wellbeing. Reflexology's ability to reduce stress and improve fertility is a fascinating topic for further research because it is based on both traditional traditions and contemporary scientific knowledge.

The Relaxation Response: The fundamental power of reflexology is its capacity to elicit the relaxation response, which is the transitional state between the body's "fight or flight" stress reaction and its "rest and digest" mode. When expert hands push on particular reflex spots, a series of physiological reactions take place. Tension dissolves, respiration deepens, and heart rate decreases. This deliberate de-stressing not only offsets the negative impacts of ongoing stress, but also fosters a conducive environment for conception.

Hormonal Harmony: The benefits of reflexology go beyond the momentary state of relaxation. The goal of practitioners' treating reproductive reflex sites is to bring hormonal balance back. The application of pressure and light manipulations to these sites may promote the release of endorphins, which are naturally occurring feel-good chemicals that reduce stress. Reproductive hormones resume their rhythmic dance when cortisol levels drop, allowing for normal ovulation, regular menstrual cycles, and a higher likelihood of pregnancy.

Improving Blood Flow: Reflexology also has the potential to increase fertility through its capacity to enhance blood circulation. Blood arteries widen and the supply of blood to the reproductive organs is maximized by activating reflex points. The uterus, fallopian tubes, and ovaries are all nourished by this enhanced circulation, which makes the environment favorable for implantation and conception.

Reducing Anxiety: Tension and anxiety fade as reflexology leads people into a calm state. The parasympathetic nervous system, which is in charge of healing processes, is highlighted. In this calm condition, libido returns, couples become more attentive to the intimate dance of conception, and psychological barriers to conception dissolve.

As a conduit to conception, reflexology empowers the journey.

In Chapter 4 of this extensive guide, the author advocates for reflexology as a tool for empowerment for couples navigating the difficult landscape of infertility, rather than just as a means of relaxation. By adopting reflexology, people start a path of self-care, integrating their body and mind, and creating an atmosphere that is favorable for conception.

Hope Despite Difficulties: There is hope that the stress-fertility link is not an insurmountable barrier. For individuals hoping to grow their family, reflexology gives promise because it can improve fertility, lower anxiety, and relieve stress. Couples that participate in this practice retake control over their reproductive journeys, supported by the idea that a holistic approach to well-being can facilitate the miracle of conception.

Collaborating with Science: The use of reflexology to increase fertility doesn't conflict with medical treatments; on the contrary, it enhances them. Reflexology can complement medical therapies by encouraging a physiologically balanced state and lowering stress levels, which may increase the effectiveness of the latter. Reflexology can be a comfort to couples using assisted reproductive technologies since it can minimize adverse effects, boost general wellbeing, and offer emotional support.

Finitude

The impact of long-term stress on reproductive function is highlighted in Chapter 4, which explores the deep relationship between stress and problems with reproduction. Reflexology shows promise as a potent strategy for reducing the negative impacts of stress by providing a comprehensive approach to relaxation, hormonal balance, and improved blood circulation. When people and couples choose reflexology, they start a life-changing process in which tension disappears, anxiety fades, and a conducive environment for conception emerges. This chapter presents readers with the therapeutic potential of reflexology and extends an invitation to engage in a harmonious relationship between science and holistic well-being, which will finally plant the seeds of renewal.

CHAPTER 5

Enhancing Blood Flow to the Reproductive Organs: Highlight the importance of proper blood circulation for reproductive health. Describe reflexology techniques that stimulate blood flow to the pelvic region, thereby improving the supply of nutrients and oxygen to reproductive organs.

Often called the life power of the body, blood flow is essential to preserving the best possible state of health and function. An essential component of reproductive health is healthy blood circulation. In addition to exploring how reflexology techniques can be used to enhance blood flow to the pelvic region, nourishing reproductive organs and encouraging fertility, this chapter looks into the significance of proper blood flow for reproductive well-being.

The Blood Flow's Significance in Reproductive Health

The effective supply of hormones, nutrients, and oxygen to all of the body's cells and tissues—including the reproductive organs—is dependent upon proper blood circulation. Enough blood flow to the testes, uterus, fallopian tubes, and ovaries is essential for fertility. Better circulation facilitates tissue healing, encourages the elimination of waste and toxins, and improves organ performance overall.

Difficulties Resulting from Inadequate Blood Flow

Reduced blood supply to the reproductive organs can cause a

number of problems with fertility. Insufficient blood circulation in females may lead to irregular menstrual cycles, diminished ovarian function, and damaged uterine lining, all of which may impact the implantation of embryos. Insufficient blood supply to the testes can impair the quality and quantity of sperm produced in men. Blood circulation in these regions can be impacted by sedentary lifestyles, stress, and medical problems, among other things.

Reflexology's Function in Improving Blood Flow

Reflexology stimulates reflex sites and encourages relaxation as two ways to improve blood flow. Tension and stress are released during relaxation, which can cause blood vessels to narrow. Reflexology stimulates certain reflex points that correspond to the reproductive system and circulatory system, which promotes vasodilation and enhances oxygenation and blood flow.

Specific Reflexology Methods for Increasing Blood Flow

1. Inverse Limb Order: This reflexology exercise concentrates on the reflex points on the foot, ankles,

and lower legs that correspond to the lower limbs. The pelvic area and reproductive organs benefit from increased blood flow to the lower body, which is brought about by stimulating these sites.

2. Pelvic Region Stimulation: By targeting reflex points in the pelvic region, reflexology techniques can help to maintain blood flow to the prostate, uterus, and ovaries. Applying light pressure to these sites improves blood vessel opening and muscle relaxation, which improves the flow of nutrients and oxygen.

3. Techniques for Lymphatic Drainage: The lymphatic system contributes to fluid balance and waste elimination. By focusing on the lymphatic reflex sites on the hands and feet, reflexology techniques can help release congestion and promote better blood flow.

How Relaxation and Stimulation Work Together

It's critical to understand that stimulation and relaxation complement one another to maximize blood flow. Tension can narrow blood arteries, but reflexology releases it by inducing relaxation through the parasympathetic nervous system reaction. In addition, reflex point activation triggers neural pathways that encourage vasodilation, which increases blood flow to the pelvic region.

A Comprehensive Strategy for Reproductive Health

Improving blood flow to the reproductive organs is important for maintaining mental and physical well-being as well as overall health. The techniques used in reflexology to induce relaxation enhance mental well-being by lowering stress and anxiety, both of which can worsen blood circulation. By cultivating this state of mind-body equilibrium, reflexology transforms into a comprehensive method for promoting reproductive health.

Result: Enriching Circulation for Reproductive Health

As we explore the many mechanisms associated with reproductive health, the importance of appropriate blood circulation becomes clear. With its ability to both relax and stimulate, reflexology is a useful tool for improving blood flow to the pelvic area, which nourishes the reproductive organs and increases fertility. Individuals and couples can take an active role in their reproductive health by incorporating targeted reflexology treatments into their daily routines. This can create an environment that is favorable to conception and the fulfillment of parenting dreams.

CHAPTER 6

**Supporting Men's Fertility
Through Reflexology: Address male
fertility issues and how reflexology
can benefit men's reproductive
health. Discuss reflexology points
that target the male reproductive
system and provide guidance for
couples to practice together.**

Men's fertility is an equally important piece of the puzzle in the complex picture of reproductive health, while women's fertility receives most of the attention. This thorough guide's sixth chapter explores male reproductive health, illuminating the many issues that men may confront and presenting reflexology as a comprehensive strategy to support and improve male fertility. By using specific reflex points and providing couples with assistance, this chapter gives people the power to take control of their reproductive health.

Managing Male Fertility Obstacles: An All-Inclusive View

A complicated interaction between physiological, hormonal, and environmental factors affects male fertility. To address these complex issues, which range from sperm quality and quantity to hormonal balance and mental well-being, a comprehensive strategy is required.

Sperm Quality and Quantity: The influence of reflexology on sperm quality and quantity is the first step towards its potential to improve male fertility. Research indicates that reflexology could play a role in sperm motility and shape, which are important aspects of a healthy conception. By focusing on particular reflex points, practitioners hope to increase blood flow to the testes, supporting these essential reproductive organs and maybe improving sperm quality and production.

Hormonal Balance: A key factor in male fertility is hormonal balance. Due to reflexology's capacity to modulate the endocrine system, hormone levels may be brought into balance. Reflex sites linked to the adrenal glands, brain, and pituitary gland can be stimulated to regulate hormone secretion and eventually support healthy reproductive function.

Reduction of Stress: Stress can have an impact on male reproductive health in the same way that it does on female fertility. Prolonged stress causes the release of cortisol, which can interfere with the creation of testosterone and upset the balance of hormones. Reflexology counteracts stress by generating relaxation, which may enhance hormone levels and general well-being.

A Therapeutic Map of the Reflex Points of Male Reproductive Health

Particular reflex sites that focus on the male reproductive system are the foundation of reflexology's strategy for promoting male fertility. This focused stimulation provides a special opening for promoting reproductive health.

Testicular Oasis: Inside the inner arch of the feet, the "Testicular Oasis" is a main reflex point related to the testes. Blood flow to the testes may improve with little pressure at this location, which could improve sperm quality and production.

Prostate Sanctuary: The prostate gland is represented by the "Prostate Sanctuary," which is situated on the inside edge of the feet. The goal of stimulating this point is to promote prostate health, which is essential to the health of the male reproductive system.

Hormonal Harmonizer: The pituitary, hypothalamus, and adrenal gland reflex points are related to hormone regulation. By balancing hormone secretion, these points can be gently manipulated to support normal reproductive function.

Recommendations for Couples: Promoting Well-Being Together

It is possible for reflexology to become a significant joint venture for couples on their conception journey, and its ability to increase male fertility is not just confined to individual practice.

Joint Practice: Reflexology is a skill that can be developed into a personal pastime for couples. By alternately pressing each other's reflex spots, partners can promote emotional support and connection in addition to physical well-being.

Open Communication: Attending reflexology together as a couple invites candid discussion about objectives, worries, and goals related to conception. By engaging in this ritual together, you can fortify your emotional connection and establish a peaceful base for your conception process.

Holistic Lifestyle Integration: One aspect of a holistic strategy for improving male fertility is reflexology. Reflexology can be combined with other lifestyle changes that couples choose to make, like eating a balanced diet, exercising regularly, and practicing relaxation techniques to reduce stress.

Finitude

This thorough guide's sixth chapter explores the field of male reproductive health and identifies the variety of obstacles that men may confront on the path to motherhood. With its holistic approach to improving male fertility through specific reflex spots and techniques for producing relaxation, reflexology emerges as a ray of hope. Individuals and couples who choose this practice go on a path of empowerment where the seeds of new life are sown and reproductive health is fostered. Through cooperative practice and honest dialogue, reflexology serves as a link between couples seeking to conceive, become one, and experience the joys of parenthood.

CHAPTER 7

Reflexology for Assisted Reproductive Techniques (ART): Explore how reflexology can complement medical interventions such as in vitro fertilization (IVF) or intrauterine insemination (IUI). Offer reflexology practices to prepare the body for these procedures and enhance their success rates.

In the field of contemporary reproductive medicine, assisted reproductive methods (ART) have completely changed the prospects for infertile couples. Intrauterine insemination (IUI) and in vitro fertilization (IVF) are two commonly used assisted reproductive technologies (ART) that provide hope to individuals trying to conceive. This chapter explores the possible synergy between ART and reflexology, looking at how both practices can increase the effectiveness of medical interventions and improve the quality of life after surgery.

Assisted   Reproductive Technologies: A Landscape

For couples struggling with infertility, assisted reproductive procedures have provided fresh avenues for hope by providing cutting-edge strategies to get through a number of obstacles to conception. During in vitro fertilization (IVF), an egg and sperm are fertilized outside the body, and the resultant embryo is then transferred into the uterus. Contrarily, IUI involves inserting prepared sperm directly into the uterus. Although these techniques have good results, they can also be physically and emotionally taxing on couples.

The Holistic Method: ART and Reflexology

Reflexology can be easily incorporated into the ART process because of its emphasis on fostering relaxation, enhancing blood circulation, and boosting general well-being. Reflexology seeks to minimize potential for failure while reducing stress and boosting emotional resilience by readying the body and mind for the operations.

Preparing for ART with Reflexology Practices

1. Relaxation Before Procedure: Couples preparing for ART procedures might reduce tension and anxiety by scheduling reflexology sessions beforehand. Reflexology techniques that focus on stress-relieving reflex points might help you relax and think more clearly and peacefully.

2. Blood Flow Enhancement: Reflexology methods intended to increase blood flow to the pelvic area might encourage the reproductive organs' supply of nutrients and oxygen, which may improve the uterine environment for the implantation of an embryo.

3. Supporting Hormonal Balance: By focusing on hormone-producing glands, reflexology techniques can help control hormone levels, which can assist create the ideal environment for follicle development and the preparation of the uterine lining.

4. Recovery Following Procedure: Reflexology has the potential to facilitate the healing process after ART operations. Sessions of gentle reflexology can support the body's natural healing processes, ease discomfort, and encourage relaxation.

Adopting Mind-Body Harmony

Reflexology and ART work together in ways that go beyond the tangible. The emotional and psychological aspects of fertility treatment are significant, and the total experience can be greatly influenced by reflexology's capacity to promote emotional balance and relaxation. Through the promotion of self-governance, self-actualization, and mind-body integration, reflexology adds a comprehensive element to the medical experience.

Interaction and Cooperation

When incorporating reflexology into their ART journey, people and couples should be open and honest with their reflexologist and medical specialists. Working together, these professionals guarantee a cohesive approach, customizing reflexology techniques to the unique requirements and schedules of the ART operations.

Final Thought: Using Reflexology to Support the ART Journey

Using ART to become a parent is a difficult and emotionally taxing process. Reflexology addresses the physical, emotional, and psychological aspects of the experience, making it a kind and encouraging companion on this journey. Reflexology can support people and couples with comfort and empowerment while enhancing the effectiveness of ART therapies by preparing the body, encouraging relaxation, and building mind-body synchronicity. The ART journey transforms into a comprehensive tapestry woven with hope, tenacity, and the possibility of fresh starts when reflexology and medical research converge.

CHAPTER 8

Lifestyle and Nutrition Tips Alongside Reflexology: Provide holistic advice by integrating reflexology with healthy lifestyle choices and nutrition. Share recommendations for optimal diets, exercise routines, and relaxation techniques to support overall fertility in conjunction with reflexology practices.

When individuals and couples traverse the complex path towards motherhood, a comprehensive strategy that integrates multiple aspects of wellbeing becomes critical. This thorough guide's eighth chapter explores the relationship between reflexology, dietary choices, and lifestyle choices, providing a detailed plan to enhance fertility. Through the integration of these factors, people may take care of their reproductive health, increase their chances of getting pregnant, and confidently and energetically take the first steps towards becoming parents.

The Influence of Holistic Health: A Comprehensive Method

There is no one element that determines fertility; rather, there is a complex interaction of environmental, psychological, and physical factors. Adopting a holistic perspective that incorporates nutrition, lifestyle decisions, and reflexology offers a multifaceted basis for promoting fertility and general well-being.

The Function of Reflexology: Reflexology is a catalyst that encourages equilibrium and activates the body's natural healing processes. It seeks to improve blood circulation, lessen stress, and balance hormone levels by focusing on particular reflex points—all important components that support reproductive health.

Lifestyle Decisions: Fertility is greatly influenced by lifestyle factors. Maintaining a healthy weight, managing stress, and exercising frequently are all factors in reproductive wellbeing. An ideal setting for conception includes taking part in joyful activities, using relaxation techniques, and making sure you get enough sleep.

Nutrition as Nourishment: The foundation of reproductive health is adequate nutrition. The body uses a balanced diet full of vital nutrients to power its complex functions, such as hormone production, the health of the egg and sperm, and the preservation of the reproductive system.

A Balanced Diet: Eating for Healthy Fertility

Eating a healthy diet is the first step towards promoting fertility. A diet high in certain nutrients improves the body's preparedness for conception and supports reproductive health.

Essential Nutrients: Include foods high in zinc, folic acid, vitamin D, antioxidants, and omega-3 fatty acids. These nutrients sustain hormone balance, aid in the generation of healthy eggs and sperm, and foster the growth of the embryo.

Colorful Variety: A rainbow of hues may be found in fruits and vegetables, which are rich in vitamins, minerals, and phytonutrients that support fertility and general health.

For Complex Carbohydrates, choose whole grains like oats, brown rice, and quinoa. These complex carbs support hormonal balance by supplying steady energy and assisting in blood sugar stabilization.

Lean Proteins: Opt for lean protein sources like fish, poultry, beans, lentils, and lean meats. Consuming enough protein maintains the health of sperm and eggs and gives reproductive cells the fundamental building blocks they need.

Hydration: Drink plenty of water and herbal teas to stay dehydrated. Staying hydrated aids in maintaining the body's physiological processes and promotes healthy production of cervical mucus.

Tranquility and Exercise: Towards Vitality

Exercise and relaxation methods are the mainstays of a comprehensive program to increase fertility.

frequent Exercise: Maintaining a healthy weight, promoting blood circulation, and balancing hormones are all benefits of frequent, moderate exercise. Walking, yoga, and swimming are a few of the easy yet powerful approaches to improve reproductive health.

Mind-Body Connection: Include mindfulness, deep breathing, and meditation as relaxing methods in your regular activities. These techniques reduce stress, establish emotional equilibrium, and improve the conditions that are favorable for conception.

Quality Sleep: Make getting 7-9 hours of sleep every night a priority. Healthy hormone balance and general wellbeing are supported by restful sleep.

Collaborating to Promote Wellbeing: A Joint Adventure

For many couples, the road to fertility is a joint one. Combining reflexology, dietary choices, and lifestyle management can be a worthwhile collaborative endeavor.

Team Approach: Adopt a collaborative strategy to improve fertility. Share nutritious meals, practice reflexology together, and encourage one another's wellness objectives.

Communication: Encourage candid discussion about difficulties, preferences, and changes in lifestyle. This mutual conversation fortifies the emotional connection and fosters a sense of oneness.

Joy and Connection: Bring happiness to the trip. Take part in things that you both enjoy doing, like cooking, going for walks, or just hanging out.

Conclusion

This comprehensive guide's Chapter 8 weaves together the domains of reflexology, diet, and lifestyle choices into a harmonious fertility support picture. Individuals and couples who adopt this comprehensive approach provide themselves the means to maximize reproductive health, improve mental well-being, and establish a conducive environment for conception. The road to motherhood is brightened with vigor, optimism, and the promise of fresh starts as reflexology triggers the body's healing reactions, lifestyle decisions support the mind-body connection, and diet supplies the building blocks of life.

9 798867 586058